For more than twenty years we have been telling
getting weaker or stronger, there's no in-between..." A simple but
consistent program is the key. Now, Tartell and Kavanau have put it
all together in a very simple, easy-to-follow, comprehensive approach
to restoring and maintaining good health. From head to toes, this
book offers the reader exercises for every joint intersection. I am
especially thrilled to see that the extremities (feet, hands and cervical
spine) are addressed, as these areas are usually forgotten in most
exercise programs. This book is a much needed addition to getting
and keeping fit. No excuses now!

> —Jim Wharton, president of Wharton Performance,
> musculoskeletal therapist, and author of *The Wharton
> Stretch Book*, *The Wharton Strength Book*, *The
> Wharton Cardio Book*, and *The Wharton Back Book*

Ted Kavanau's funny and plaintive introduction to this book alone is
worth the price of the book. The "in-bed" exercises are simply
presented with self-explanatory photos. The exercises themselves would
seem to be good for reducing stress. New reports indicate that
exercise before sleeping may actually help induce a calm and restful
sleep. These exercises are ideally suited to that purpose.

> —Rochelle Medici, Ph.D., neurophysiologist in private
> practice in San Marino, CA

This book is a good start for getting fit in a holistic way. It can lead
one to the next step in the world of fitness safely.

> —Catherine Lloyd, coordinator of the Group Fitness
> Program at Marymount Manhattan College and a
> certified personal trainer

Get Fit in Bed provides exercises to improve recovery and help maintain strength. All of us are temporarily able-bodied and one never knows when one may experience a life altering injury. This book provides an option for anyone less mobile to stay fit. As I tell my nursing students, mobility is essential for life and starting with bed mobility is crucial. Get Fit in Bed should be in every nursing home and at the bedside of anyone who is bed-bound for any reason.

> —Sheree Loftus Fader, MSN, APRN, BC, CRRN, gerontologist, geriatric nurse practitioner, and certified physical rehabilitation nurse

Try this routine; it may give you startling results.

> —Harold Rubin, licensed psychologist in Massachusetts

When I first heard of our attempt to reach the moon, I said, 'Yeah, maybe we can do that.' When I heard of our attempt to get live pictures from Mars, I said, 'Yeah, maybe we can do that.' When I saw a book entitled Get Fit in Bed, I said, 'Get outta here!' And I got the third one wrong. Tartell and Kavanau have given us a valid and valuable road map to getting a great workout without even getting up. Joy will be felt. Health will be ours. Lives will be saved.

> —Barry Farber, nationally syndicated radio talk host on the Talk Radio Network

get fit
in Bed

Tone Your Body & Calm Your Mind from the Comfort of Your Bed

GENIE TARTELL, DC, RN • TED KAVANAU

New Harbinger Publications, Inc.

Publisher's Note

This publication is designed to provide accurate and authoritative information in regard to the subject matter covered. It is sold with the understanding that the publisher is not engaged in rendering psychological, financial, legal, or other professional services. If expert assistance or counseling is needed, the services of a competent professional should be sought.

Distributed in Canada by Raincoast Books.

Copyright © 2006 by Ted Kavanau and Genie Tartell, DC, RN
New Harbinger Publications, Inc.
5674 Shattuck Avenue
Oakland, CA 94609
www.newharbinger.com

Cover design by Amy Shoup
Cover photo by Pixland/Index Stock
Interior photography by Laura Rose
Photo post production by Carrie Villines
Text design by Michele Waters
Acquired by Tesilya Hanauer
Edited by Brady Kahn

Printed in the United States of America

Library of Congress Cataloging-in-Publication Data

Tartell, Genie.
  Get fit in bed : tone your body & calm your mind from the comfort of your bed / Genie Tartell and Ted Kavanau.
       p. cm.
   ISBN-13: 978-1-57224-460-3
   ISBN-10: 1-57224-460-7
  1. Exercise. I. Kavanau, Ted. II. Title.
   RA781.T228 2006
   613.7'1—dc22
                            2006014696

08 07 06

10 9 8 7 6 5 4 3 2 1

First printing

Contents

ACKNOWLEDGMENTS

The authors want to thank Margaret Kavanau, Ph.D. (psychologist) for reviewing and giving her advice about improving the manuscript.

The authors also want to thank Steve Bauman for his patient and detailed help in all the phases of getting this book completed. We hope he uses the exercises to help calm himself down after all his stressful efforts on our behalf and also to keep himself fit, something his wife, Dr. Genie Tartell, would certainly appreciate.

INTRODUCTION

TED KAVANAU: From the Founding of CNN to Getting Fit in Bed

I had no idea how good the results were going to be when I started exercising in bed or that there might one day be a book about it. I needed some exercise and had not found a regimen I could stick with. I also didn't like getting down on the floor, especially one that was carpeted. It seems I have some sensitivity to dust, and in my mind, no amount of vacuuming a carpet will really do the job. I had visited a few health clubs, but their hard sells and lengthy contracts worried me. So I never signed up. There was also a drastic financial circumstance that contributed to my choosing to exercise in bed. How I reacted may seem a little extreme to you, but I assure you that it all happened just the way I am going to relate it.

I had been working in TV news for decades, mostly in management at stations in New York City. Sometimes I did some reporting on the air. A couple of professional high points came toward the end of my career. I was one of a small team of executives who founded CNN. As the network's first senior producer, I designed and supervised the editorial system for the world's first twenty-four-hour TV news organization. I later created and ran Headline News, CNN's second twenty-four-hour TV news network. Some might say my greatest contribution to the news business happened when, on an impulse, I asked a young desk assistant to cohost with me on a late-night CNN program called *Real Pictures*. That cohost has continued to do well in her career. Her name is Katie Couric.

During my career, successes like CNN have been interspersed with very unpleasant failures. A social scientist's graph of my career would look like a child's drawing of mountains, several very high peaks with very low valleys in between. Creating and maintaining a success was challenge and stress enough, while living through failures and the memory of them was far more stressful.

So, I was relieved when I retired from the news business, leaving all those pressures with my health seemingly intact. I was able to live reasonably well with the money I had carefully squirreled away during my career. Any "work" in retirement consisted of writing indignant Letters to the Editor and e-mailing copies of articles that interested me to friends and former colleagues. I also did some unpaid appearances on syndicated radio, along with a few on national cable news, mostly commenting on somebody else's problems and thinking how fortunate I was to no longer be a potential target myself.

Just when I thought I had my retirement comfortably structured, I was hit with some serious personal difficulties and had to spend a lot of my savings. Trying to find a way to pay all the incoming bills, I began investing (okay . . . gambling) heavily in the stock market. After a year or two, almost all my savings were gone or, more accurately, in the hands of shrewder traders. I needed a major attitude adjustment to live with the problems I was facing, which now included this significant financial loss. All this called for a much more modest lifestyle, which brought on what I call my "Monkish Period."

I moved from my multiroomed high-rise apartment to a much less expensive place. Cynics might describe it as a basement while I choose to see it as a charming, compact garden apartment. For reasons that psychologists may plumb, I decided that toughening myself in the face of adversity required getting rid of my comfortable bed. So, I gave it away to someone who undoubtedly did not believe in the efficacy of sleep-time suffering.

My new apartment came with a folding couch that had been left behind when my new landlady's daughter moved to another town. I thought it not suitable for the ascetic rigors I had chosen (though if you have ever slept on a folding couch, you know it is no bed of roses). Instead, I purchased a very simple folding cot, the kind with a one-inch mattress and single layer of springs. These cots may be fine for camping, or for a guest (especially if you don't want that person to stay over again). But, unless they're for temporary use or you're seeking some higher philosophical purpose, I would not recommend them.

During this same period, I decided to try to make some money in independent TV production. Karate movies were all the rage, and I had an idea to produce a pilot video for cable TV that would incorporate karate movements into a daily exercise program. Through a friend, I met a karate instructor who could host the show, and the three of us actually produced the pilot program. Unfortunately, we discovered that marketing is a totally separate skill from producing, and it seemed my friend and I totally lacked the marketing gene. So, the pilot program remained in a drawer and I returned to sleeping on my cot and, by punishing my body, reforming my inner being. (It should be noted that a few years later, Billy Blanks' Tae Bo exercise video became a raging financial success. Clearly, either Billy, or someone in his employ, had the marketing gene we lacked.)

There was perhaps a happy ending of sorts to this entrepreneurial effort, especially for the karate instructor. He, being of sound instincts, benefited from the unsold TV program by successfully using a copy to impress potential girlfriends. He also derived at least some income from our relationship when he invited me to join his karate school, which had a reasonable monthly membership fee and no contracts. Out of shape physically as well as mentally, I joined his school (or "dojo" in karate-speak), becoming, by many decades, his oldest student. Karate, in addition to teaching self-defense and being good exercise, is said to improve you as a person. That latter concept seemed to fit well with my necessary pursuit of modesty in all matters, something which certainly included my cot with its one-inch mattress.

Unfortunately, or fortunately in a yin/yang kind of way, I was very much out of shape, tired rapidly, and ached after the rigorous karate training. I figured I better do some exercising in preparation for the exercise in karate class. I thought maybe I could do it at home, but there was a lot of dust-exuding carpet on the floor there. After a restless night, tossing and turning very carefully on my narrow cot, I awoke to what Zen masters might agree was a burst of enlightenment. The answer to avoiding the carpet would be exercising on the cot.

So, I started to experiment on the cot by doing some full sit-ups. Doing sit-ups is a vigorous exercise, and after I did a few, there was a sudden twanging sound. A cot spring had snapped. I repaired the gap left under the mattress by replacing the broken spring with a bungee cord, hooking the ends of the bungee to other springs on the cot. Even with the hook ends pointing toward the floor, however, they created small, uncomfortable bulges I could feel through the thin mattress. I dropped the sit-ups from my regimen and continued with my experiments. I tried movements from every exercise discipline I had known, as well as movements I thought up. Of course, in the history of the world, there is probably nothing new in exercise. Qi gong, for example, which is a collection of ancient Chinese exercise, is said to have thousands of movements. Every time one of the exercises I tried caused another broken spring, which was frequent, I added a bungee cord and dropped that exercise from my practice.

Months passed, and sleep and exercise on the cot became more and more uncomfortable. At the same time, I was developing a repertoire of exercises that were easier on the cot and easy to do. Then years passed, and the cot became supported almost completely by crisscrossed bungees. Finally, serious discomfort trumped philosophy, and I moved to the folding couch.

By then I had developed a routine. I did a certain number of exercises on my back, then on my right side, followed by a repeat of those exercises on my left side. Lastly, I did exercises while facing down on the cot. I also had developed a particular sequence for doing the movements, so that earlier exercises were a warm-up for later ones that required a little more effort. Rather than moving slowly through all the exercises, I started speeding up some of them. Others I did more slowly and with fewer repetitions. Surprisingly, even when going through the whole series of exercises, I found myself relaxed, and almost always free of perspiration.

Some other benefits from exercising in bed came as a surprise. When I did it in the mornings, I became both relaxed and invigorated. I also tried exercising when I went to bed at night. I know that many doctors insist that exercising close to bedtime keeps you awake, but I found just the opposite often happened. Rather than toss and turn at bedtime with concerns from the day, I did some or all of the exercises and frequently found myself calm and quickly asleep. I also experimented with exercising if I awoke in the middle of the night. Restless thoughts could keep me from falling back to sleep, so I used that "up" time to do the exercises. Focusing on the repetitions of these gentle movements in bed calmed my thoughts, and I often found myself soon asleep again.

I noticed that the exercises created a good foundation for other athletic activity. For example, I always found it effective to do the exercises in bed on mornings before going to weekend karate sparring sessions. The exercises limbered my body and, as just one specific example, strengthened me against karate kicks to my stomach.

In my sixties, I actually entered a karate tournament in Las Vegas. My dojo associates were going there to fight and my instructor invited me along to watch the matches and to enjoy the city with them. Once there, to his dismay, I insisted on signing up for the competition. I am told it was a good fight while it lasted, but I didn't get beyond the first round, since my opponent had a better kick and was carrying forty or so fewer years than I.

I persisted in karate classes for about eight years. Whether recognizing skills I had developed, or just in sympathy for my long effort, the instructor finally awarded me a black belt. Boxing is part of the training in our karate style, so I thought I would put that part to a test. In April of 2005, at age seventy-two, I fought three rounds in the monthly White Collar Sparring competition at Gleason's Gym in Brooklyn. That's the gym where Hilary Swank learned boxing for the film *Million Dollar Baby*. There was no winner in the match. Just getting in and out of the ring on my feet was an accomplishment. Several left hooks to my head will serve as a reminder (if I ever decide to get back in the ring) to keep my hands up and practice more ducking.

It was only a few years ago that I decided to write a book about my experiences exercising in bed, believing it could be useful to others of all ages, from top athletes to those rehabilitating from injury or illness. I approached Marianne Strong, a prominent literary agent in New York City, who suggested finding a coauthor with medical expertise in this specific area, who would know what worked, what didn't, and what cautions should be observed.

I was fortunate to be acquainted with someone we both considered ideal, Dr. Genie Tartell, a nationally known Manhattan-based chiropractor who has appeared on ABC television's *The View* program. Dr. Tartell cowrote this book and is shown in all the photographs. She includes, in the following pages, her experience doing the exercises herself and having some of her chiropractic patients try them.

GENIE TARTELL: From Athletes to the Homebound, Healing Through Fitness

I had always wanted to write a book to share my knowledge of health maintenance. I have been a health care professional for over twenty-five years. Initially, I was a public health nurse working with homebound patients who were newly discharged from the hospital or homebound because of chronic debilitating illnesses. I monitored their recovery and established personal protocols to help with their adaptation to their limitations. Most of the time, this included diet and exercise counseling. My hospital experience was with chronic and, then, intensive-care cardiac patients. Again, diet and exercise were the foundations of their recovery and, in many cases, their survival.

I discovered chiropractic care to treat a personal injury, was amazed by the results, and decided to become a chiropractor. I am presently a certified chiropractic sports practitioner with certificates in chiropractic acupuncture and the Whartons' sports exercise program. My practice encompasses all my basic philosophies about health. A healthy body requires adequate nutrition, a good mental outlook, and appropriate, frequent body movements to maintain functionality. My practice presently treats a broad population of individuals from newborns to the quite elderly. They include professional dancers, world-class runners, and aerobic competitors, many of whom I have treated for the entire twenty years I've been in practice. This gives me the unique experience of seeing the changes aging has on the body and how a regular exercise program can slow down that process.

I have known Ted for many years and have a great deal of respect for his past accomplishments. He and my husband worked together in broadcast news in New York. Additionally, he is one of the most fit seventy-plus-year-olds I know. He claimed that this series of exercises was the foundation of his workout and, to boot, if done at night it induced sleep. My initial response was to question the concept of exercising in bed, especially before attempting to sleep. Some also assume that a bed is an unsupportive surface, and that exercise should not be done before bedtime. So, I decided to implement the program on my own. I performed the exercises for fifteen days, on the bed, before sleep, and indeed they worked remarkably. My back showed no signs of strain, and my sleep was greatly improved. I looked for research that related to Ted's concept. On January 24, 2006 the New York Times did an article citing a study published in 1998 by the journal, Physiology and Behavior that agreed with the experience we had doing "Get Fit In Bed" exercises before sleep. A group of college students were reported, to have exercised moderately for about an hour on two separate nights, in one case ninety minutes before bedtime and in the other thirty minutes before bed. Researchers found that the exercise had no significant effects on the amount of time the subjects needed to fall asleep, nor did it negatively affect the quality of their sleep. The Times reported that, "Other studies have had similar findings." In fact the Times quoted one widely published researcher in the field, Dr. Shawn

D. Youngstedt, saying he, "... believes that exercise before bed can actually promote sleep, easing anxiety and raising body temperature. But the effects vary from person to person ..." In evaluating the system even further, I then began incorporating these exercises into my patients' rehabilitation regime. They reported increased range of motion and diminished pain in the affected area, with an increased rate of recovery. I recalled the exercise programs I had used many years ago with bed-bound patients, in order to reduce their risk of blood clots, bone and muscle-mass loss, and pneumonia. Those exercises, done in bed three to four times daily, had produced consistently positive results. I started incorporating modifications into Ted's regime for my patients who have chronic skeletal or medical problems. Again the results were impressive. We began working together on the best way to structure the system for those outside my practice. Hence this book, including the specific modifications for those who require them.

As with any exercise program, your general health must be evaluated.

- Have you ever participated in an exercise program? If so, what were your restrictions?
- Are you currently on any medications that affect your coordination, mental alertness, or muscle strength?
- What, if any, are your flexibility restrictions?
- Do you have breathing problems?

If so, these issues should be addressed with your health care professional before you begin this or any other exercise program. Once cleared for activity, you can join this pleasant process for increased health and natural well-being.

Whatever your level of fitness, we recommend that you start the program in sequence and follow the level of repetitions suggested. The exercises should be performed with deliberate and mindful motion. Remain aware of which body part is active; this helps you to establish neuromuscular control and coordination. **If you experience any strain or discomfort in a body part while doing an exercise, stop that particular exercise and modify the movement. If the episode occurs again, I suggest eliminating that particular exercise from the sequence.** I recommend increasing the repetitions by five each week. Ted performs about fifty repetitions of most of the exercises while I have built up to between twenty-five and thirty. Again, this is a self-motivated program allowing the user to be in full control. Included are the concepts of Pilates, which will build core stability and strengthen the abdominal, gluteal, low-back, and pelvic regions. These movements will stabilize the spinal column, reducing the work your body needs to do to move through space, as well as helping to reduce the risk of low-back injuries. The yoga exercises function to relax the mind and body. They too function to build core stability and flexibility. Postures like the bridge and cobra are wonderful for enhancing the body's form and function. Yoga breathing relieves stiffness in the body and energizes the nervous system. Martial arts builds strength, core stamina, coordination, and patterned breathing. The karate-style snap kick exercise is a perfect example.

You will see that we have structured the exercises into body-position sections. First on the back, then side to side, and finally finishing on the stomach. We did this for ease of remembering and consistency. However, you will notice that the greatest percentage of the exercises are done while on your back. Therefore, if you are short on time or on wind, the series performed while on your back can be quite a substantial workout in itself. After a few days of working out, you'll notice an increase in balance, tone, and muscle strength. As with so many things, consistency is the key to results.

CHAPTER ONE

HOW TO USE THIS BOOK

As you work your way through these exercises in bed, we encourage you to do them in the order shown. This book introduces a complete exercise system in which the flow of movements has a certain physical logic. Earlier, smaller movements build tone, strength, and flexibility for later, broader movements. For example, the simple arm stretches done early in chapter 2, as you exercise on your back, help build toward the more vigorous punching-type movements later in that same chapter.

You'll start in chapter 2 with the sequence of exercises on your back and then move on to exercises on your right side (chapter 3), exercises on your left side (chapter 4), and exercises on your stomach (chapter 5). At the end of each of these chapters, you will find a list of the exercises that were just covered. A list of all the exercises appears in chapter 6. These lists will help you remember the order to complete them in.

To do the exercises, simply follow the instructions, using the photographs of the positions to help guide you. Before you begin, however, we've attempted to answer some questions that you may have.

Are There Any Special Breathing Techniques?

When first starting to do the exercises, especially if you are not in good physical condition or are recuperating from injury or illness, it's best to start slowly and practice deep and even breathing. As you speed up the movements, adding repetitions, normal breathing works well.

Several yoga-based exercises in the book (the cobra, locust, modified bow) are best always done with slower, deeper breathing.

You should never feel light-headed during this program. If so, stop until you are feeling well enough to continue.

How Many Repetitions Should You Do?

In the beginning, avoid doing too many repetitions or doing them too rapidly. Each exercise includes a suggestion for how many repetitions you should do as you start out. As you become more physically conditioned, you can increase the number. For some exercises, you may build up to fifty repetitions. For others, like the slower yoga-based movements, you may never want to do more than five repetitions.

How Do You Keep the Movement Count?

Each complete move of an arm (as in an arm stretch, up and then down) or leg (as in a leg lift, up and then down) or an upper body move (as in a stomach crunch) counts for one movement. A more complicated exercise, for example, a leg kick that requires a few moves (raising your knee toward your stomach before you raise your shin up for the kick, then reversing the process and bringing the leg back down to the bed), still counts as just one movement.

Keeping count also distracts the mind, and in that way the exercise becomes a moving meditation, helping to calm you.

How Often Should You Exercise?

We suggest that you go through all the movements at least three times a week, even if you don't go through the whole sequence each time. That way, your body maintains the toning and strengthening benefits that you have already established. As you progress in repetitions, you are likely to see gains not only physically but also mentally. These repetitious movements in bed, in our experience, actually bring a calming effect. That's why maintaining your body at a reasonably toned level makes a lot of sense.

Should You Do All the Exercises Each Time?

You can decide each time you exercise whether you want to go through all the exercises in the book or only some of them. While we encourage you to do all the exercises each time—doing so should take only fifteen to twenty minutes once you are familiar with them—you can choose to complete just one sequence of exercises at a time. You'll get many of the benefits of exercising in bed whether or not you do all the exercises each time.

Let's suppose you decide to exercise on your back. If so, we suggest you go through the whole sequence of those movements. Later during the day, you may decide to do more exercising in bed. You might then exercise on your sides. Maybe later on, you can complete the exercises on your stomach. Again, it's a good idea to follow the exercises in the order shown and to complete each sequence that you start. We think that you will soon come to appreciate the benefits of doing these exercises in bed and you will want to do them, or some sequence(s) of them, more often than not.

What Time Is Best for Doing the Exercises?

There is no best time. You can do these exercises whenever you feel like it: in the morning, afternoon, evening, before going to bed, or even when you wake up in the middle of the night. You will discover how you react to doing the exercises during any period in the twenty-four-hour cycle.

What If You Feel Tired, Out of Breath, or Get a Cramp?

If you feel tired, stop and rest for as long as it takes to recover the energy to continue. The same is true if you find yourself out of breath. If you get a cramp, relax until the cramp goes away. If you can't continue with the same exercise, move on to the next one.

When and How Should You Use Your Pillow?

A pillow is used to relieve strain on the lower back, neck, or knee areas. If you have problems in these regions, use your pillow as support by placing it as shown in the photos. The book also notes those exercises where using a pillow is especially advised. Otherwise, using or not using a pillow is your choice. We have found that having a pillow under the head while exercising on the back works well and feels comfortable, but on the sides or on the stomach, it may not.

How Can You Make This a No-Stress Workout?

Avoid making the exercises a competition with yourself. Try to enjoy your time doing these movements in your bed. If you can't match the exercise positions shown in the photos, don't worry about it. Just do the movements as best you can. Additional muscle tone and flexibility will come in time, but even if it happens slowly, you will get physical benefits and more calmness of mind by doing only what you comfortably can do.

Now, let's get started.

CHAPTER TWO

EXERCISES ON YOUR BACK

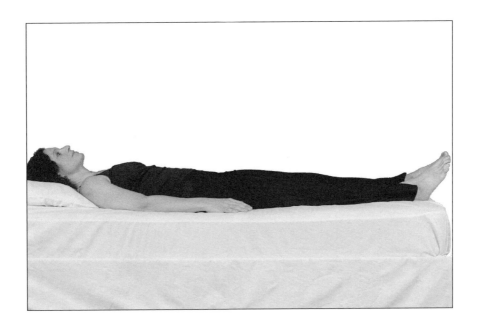

RAISING YOUR HEAD

- Lie with your arms at your sides and your legs flat on the bed.

- Bring your chin to your chest, raising your head and avoiding any strain on your neck. Lift your head slowly.

- Hold for two seconds.

- Lower your head back on the bed for two seconds.

- Repeat five times.

TIP: *Try to follow the breathing techniques recommended on page 12. You may find using a pillow to be more comfortable while exercising on your back.*

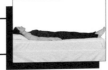

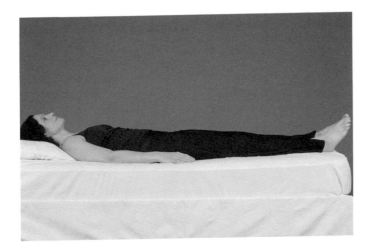

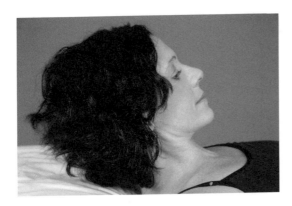

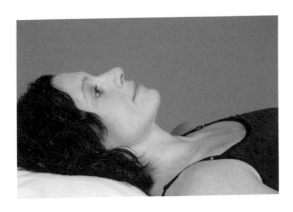

ALTERNATE LEG LENGTHENER

- With hips and legs flat on the bed, stretch the right leg forward from your hips through the heel of your right foot, keeping your leg straight.

- Bring your right leg back to the starting position.

- Do this same movement with your left leg.

- Repeat five times with each leg, alternating the leg movements for a total count of ten movements.

TIP: *Each forward stretching move may be very small, but you will feel it. (The movement is somewhat exaggerated in the photos for demonstration purposes.)*

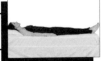

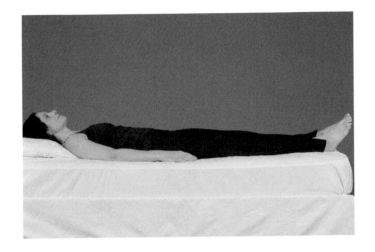

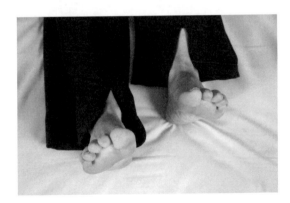

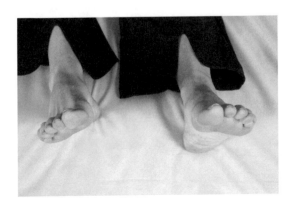

ANKLE CIRCLES

- Make circles with both feet simultaneously. (One will probably move in a clockwise direction while the other moves in a counterclockwise direction.)

- Repeat ten times.

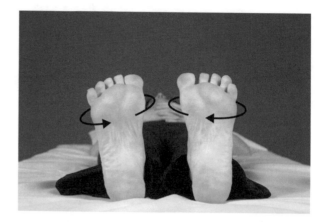

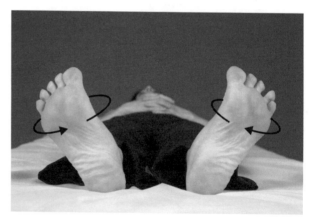

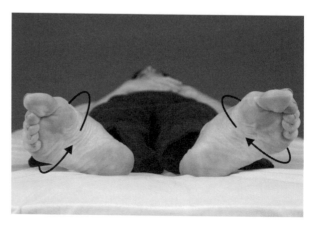

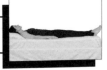

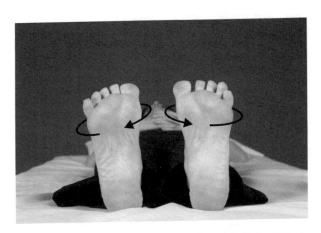

- Circle your feet in the opposite direction.

- Repeat ten times.

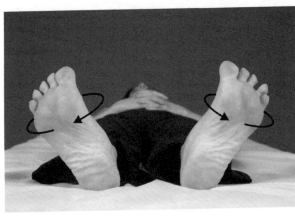

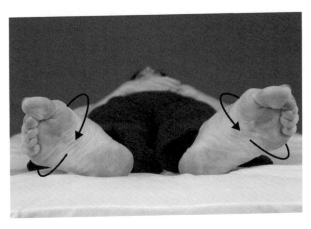

POINTING FEET AND TOES

- Simultaneously point both your feet and toes toward the bottom of your bed, flexing and extending your feet.

- Hold for two seconds.

- Point feet and toes toward your head.

- Hold for two seconds.

- Repeat ten times.

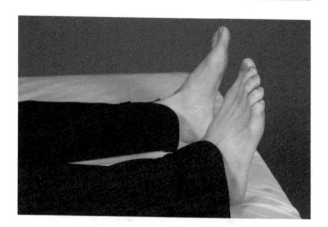

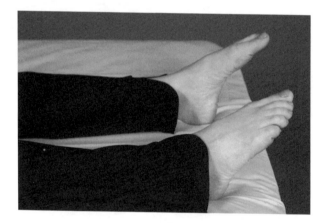

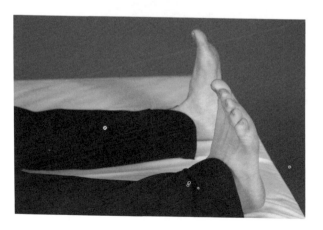

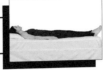

Dr. Genie's Modification:

Use a pillow under your knees to reduce the strain on your lower back.

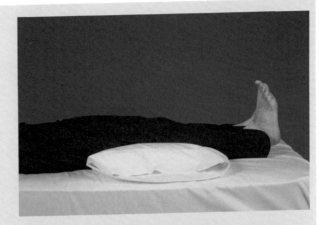

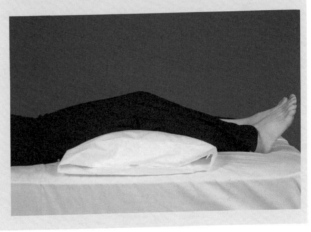

TOE WIGGLING

- Simultaneously wiggle the toes of both feet.

- Repeat fifteen times.

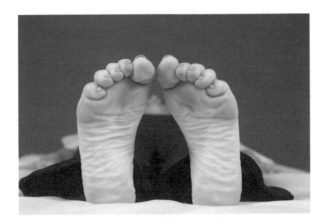

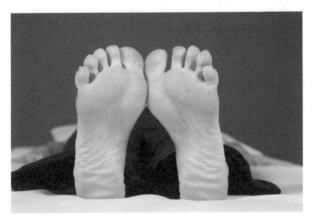

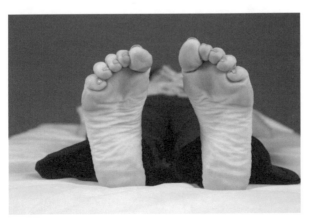

KNEE BOUNCE, THIGH FLEX

- Lie with your arms at your sides and legs flat on the bed.

- Lift both knees off the bed slightly.

- Tighten your thigh muscles and press your knees into the mattress.

- Repeat five times.

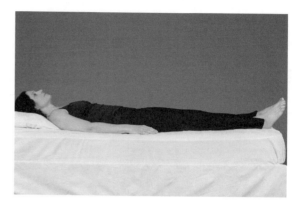

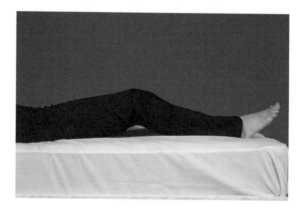

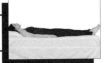

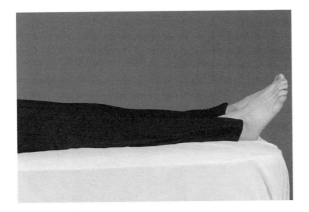

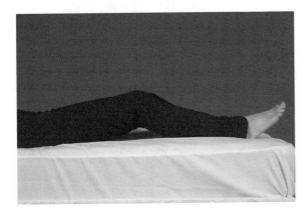

Dr. Genie's Modification:

Putting a pillow under the knees helps to reduce the strain in the lower back and knees.

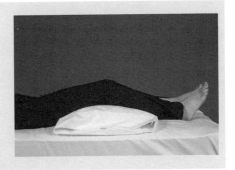

HIPS SIDE TO SIDE

- Keeping your hips flat on the bed, rock them sideways back and forth.

- Repeat five times to each side.

  TIP: *Don't jerk or overextend the movement of your hips.*

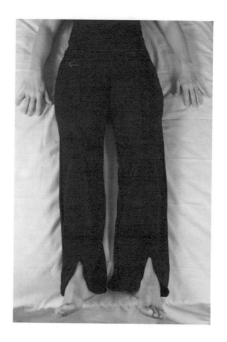

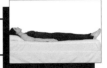

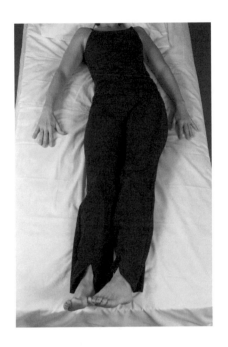

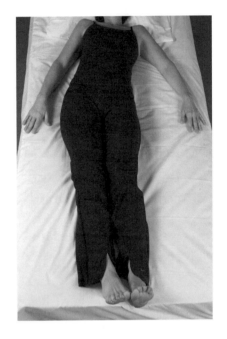

Dr. Genie's Modification:

Bend knees slightly and then move knees from side to side. Repeat five times to each side.

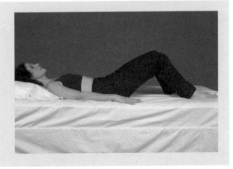

ARMS-SHOULDERS SEESAW

- Start with your arms straight at your sides, with your shoulders in a comfortable position.

- Slide your right arm down toward your right foot.

- Bring it back, raising your shoulder toward your head.

- As you bring your right arm back, slide your left arm down toward your left foot. Then bring it back up while the right arm goes downward again.

- Repeat five times on each side for a total count of ten repetitions.

TIP: *Avoid pulling downward with your hand. Instead, slide each shoulder and arm together, so your shoulders move up and down like a seesaw.*

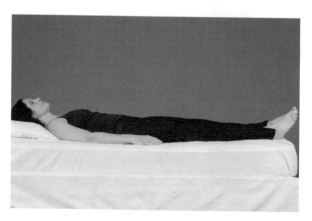

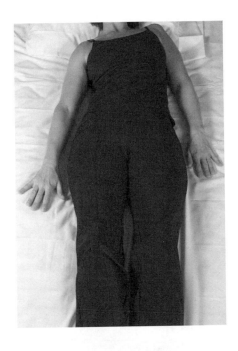

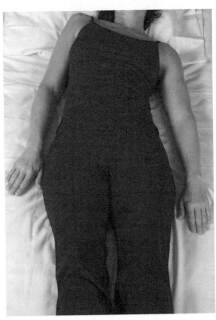

ARMS TOWARD HEADBOARD

- Start with your arms overhead, resting on the bed.

- Alternate stretching each of your arms back toward the headboard of your bed or toward the wall behind you.

- Repeat five times on each side for a total count of ten repetitions.

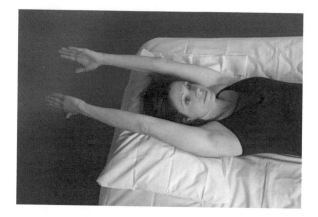

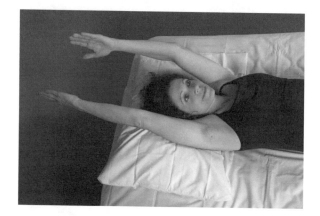

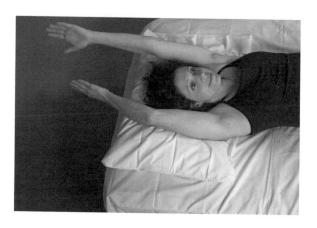

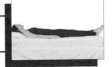

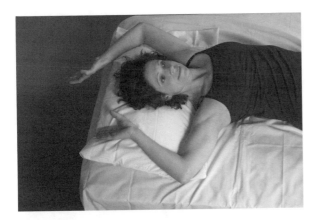

TIP: *If the headboard or wall is too close, bend your arms.*

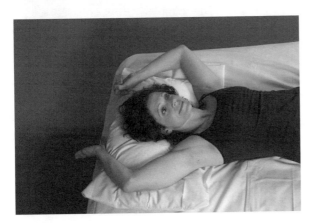

ARMS TOWARD CEILING

- Start with your arms upward, pointing toward the ceiling.

- Alternate stretching each arm toward the ceiling.

- Repeat five times with each arm for a total count of ten repetitions.

    TIP: *Avoid yanking your arm. Raise arms and shoulders together toward the ceiling.*

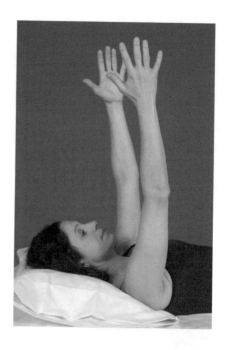

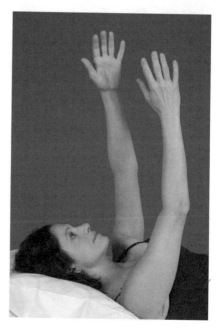

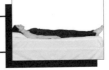

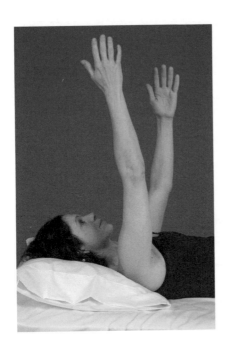

WRIST CIRCLES

- Start with your arms upward, pointing toward the ceiling.

- With hands lightly clenched, make circles with both wrists simultaneously. (One will probably move in a clockwise direction while the other moves in a counter-clockwise direction.)

- Repeat ten times.

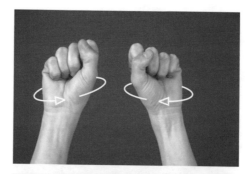

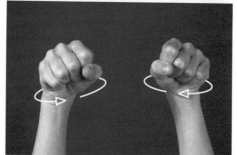

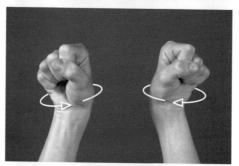

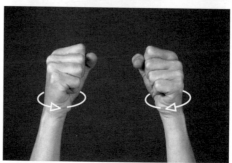

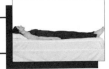

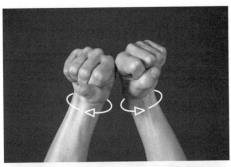

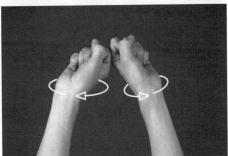

- Circle your wrists in the opposite direction.

- Repeat ten times.

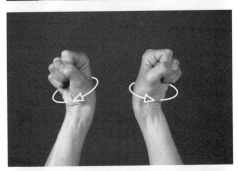

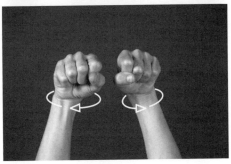

FINGER FLING

- Start with your arms upward, pointing toward the ceiling.

- Close both your hands lightly into fists.

- Gently fling your fingers outward, stretching open your hands.

- Repeat ten times.

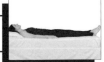

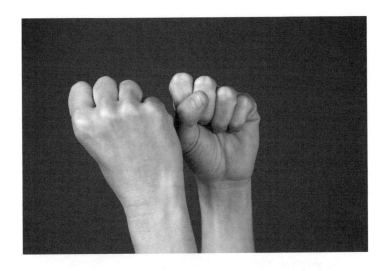

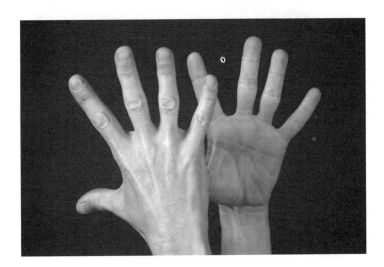

MINIMAL CRUNCH

- With arms at your sides, inhale as you tighten your stomach muscles.

- Exhale as you raise your head and shoulders very slightly off the bed (perhaps an inch or so).

- Hold for a second or two.

- Return head and shoulders to bed.

- Repeat five times.

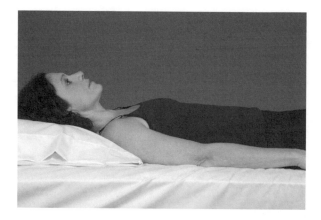

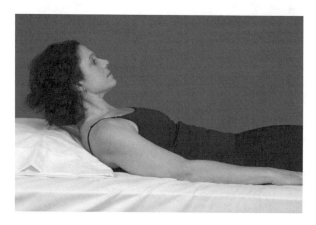

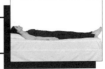

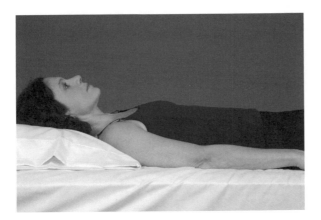

Dr. Genie's Modification:

If you have neck problems, avoid raising your head and shoulders. Just tightening your stomach muscles will condition them.

43

MODIFIED PELVIC TILT

- Keeping your hips and legs flat on the bed, tighten your buttocks, and groin muscles to raise your pelvic area slightly upward. Hold for a second or two.

- Return pelvic area to bed.

- Repeat five times.

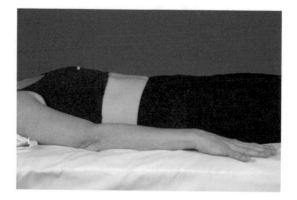

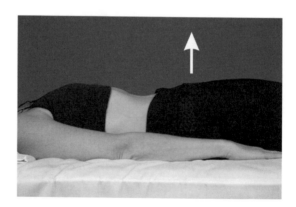

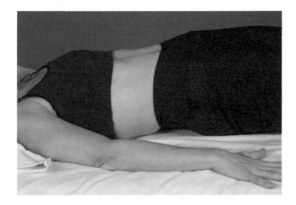

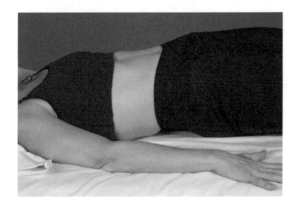

Dr. Genie's Modification:

If you have back problems, bend your knees and keep feet flat on the bed as you do this exercise.

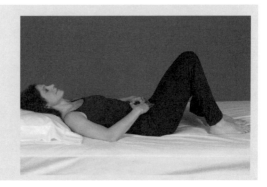

THE BRIDGE

- Start with your knees bent and feet flat on the bed. Place your arms at your sides.

- Tighten the buttock muscles as you lift your pelvis toward the ceiling until pelvis is in line with your thighs.

- Come back down to the bed gently.

- Repeat five times.

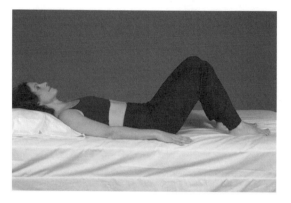

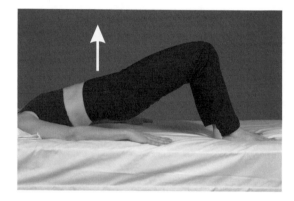

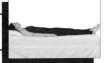

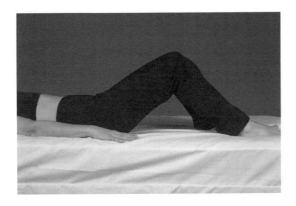

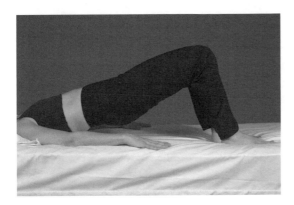

Dr. Genie's Modification:

If you have back or knee problems, place your feet further from your buttocks and raise your pelvis only to a comfortable level.

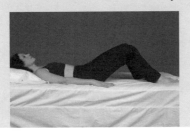

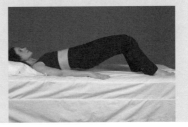

KARATE SNAP KICK—LEFT LEG

- Lie with your arms at your sides and legs flat on the bed.

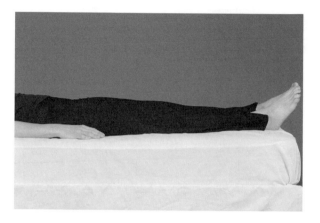

- Lift your left leg, bending your knee at a right angle. (Your foot should be pointing toward the foot of the bed.)

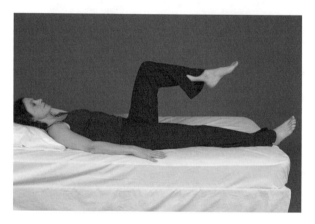

- Kick your left leg upward toward the ceiling until it is as straight as is comfortable for you.

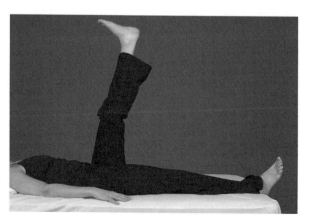

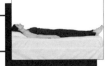

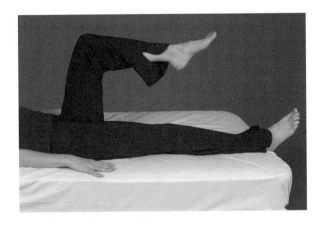

- Return left leg to the bent-knee position.

- Straighten your leg as you return it to the bed.

- Repeat five times.

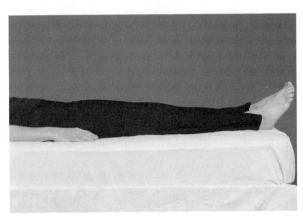

KARATE SNAP KICK—RIGHT LEG

- Lie with your arms at your sides and legs flat on the bed.

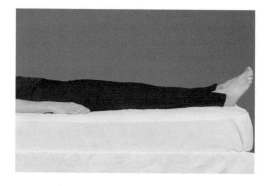

- Lift your right leg, bending your knee at a right angle. (Your foot should be pointing toward the foot of the bed.)

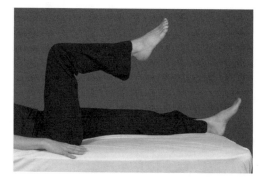

- Kick your right leg upward toward the ceiling until it is as straight as is comfortable for you.

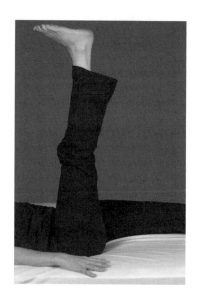

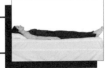

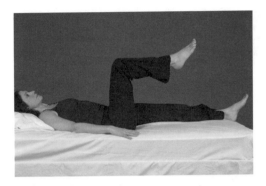

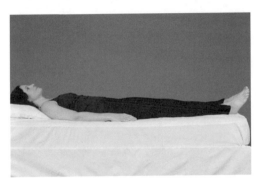

- Return right leg to the bent-knee position.

- Straighten your leg as you return it to the bed.

- Repeat five times.

THE CRUNCH

- Start with your knees bent and feet flat on the bed. Place your arms at your sides.

- Bring your knees up toward your chest.

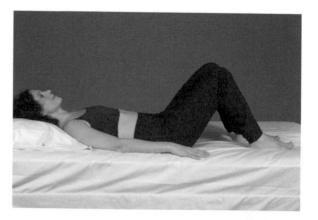

- With your hands reaching toward your knees, use your stomach muscles (not pulling with your neck) to bring your upper body closer to your knees.

- Lower your upper body halfway down toward the bed.

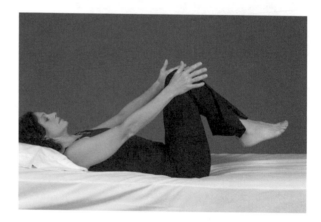

- Again, move your upper body toward your knees.

- Repeat five times.

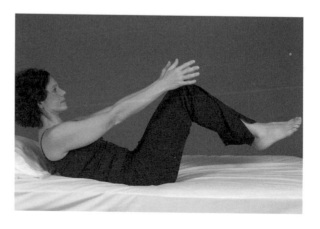

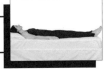

Dr. Genie's Modification:

Bring your feet up a few inches from the bed, bending your knees, and then lower them back down again.

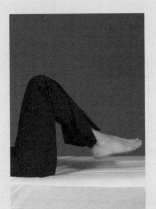

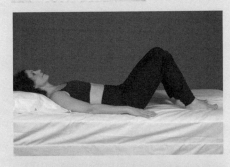

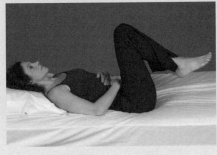

THE ARM-LEG SWITCH

- Extend both arms across one side of your body and, while moving, bend your knees in the opposite direction.

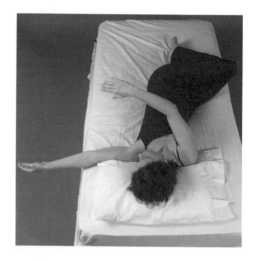

- Then switch, reversing the direction of both arms and knees.

- Repeat this movement six times.

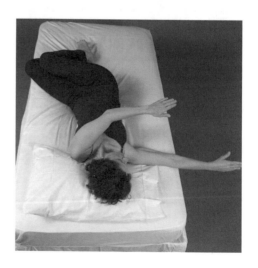

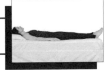

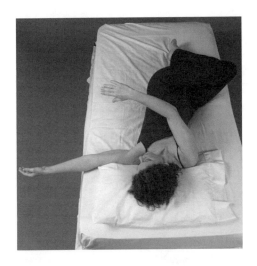

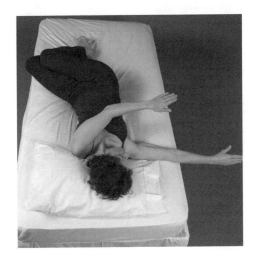

55

THE ELBOW-KNEE PISTON

- Raise your knees toward your head as you bring your upper body toward your knees.

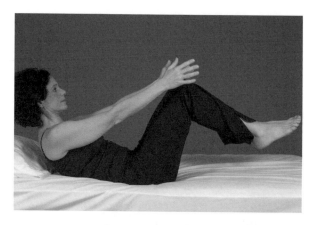

- Bend your elbows and point them at the corresponding knee (left to left, right to right).

- In alternating motions, bring your left elbow and your right knee toward each other and then, as you move your left elbow and right knee away, bring your right elbow and your left knee toward each other. (This becomes a continuous pumping motion.)

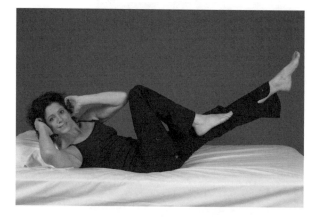

- Repeat this movement six times.

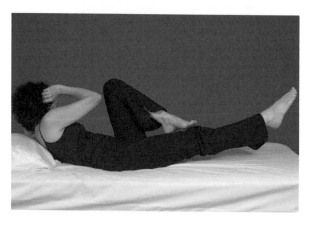

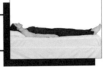

Dr. Genie's Modification:

Raise your upper body and then gently roll both knees from side to side, from the hips rather than the waist.

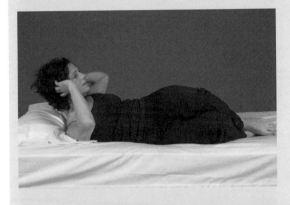

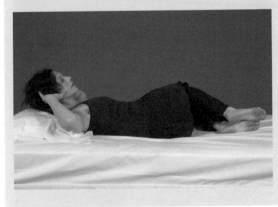

ROUNDHOUSE LEG KICK—RIGHT LEG

- Lie with your arms at your sides and legs flat on the bed.

- Bend your right knee, keeping your foot flat on the bed, and then straighten your leg up toward the ceiling.

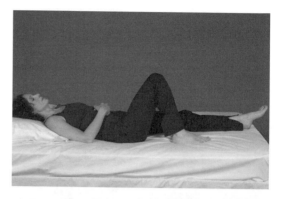

- Lower the leg across your body toward the left side of the bed, toes touching the bed if possible. (Let your hips and shoulders rotate to help your leg cross your body.)

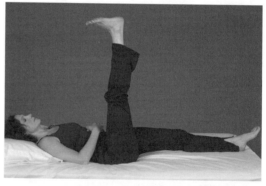

- Return your leg, hips, and shoulders to the starting position by bringing your leg back straight up toward the ceiling, then down on the bed.

- Repeat three times.

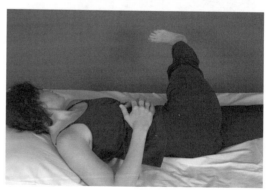

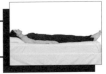

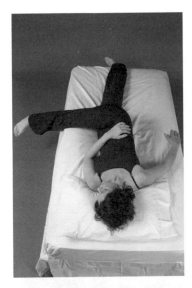

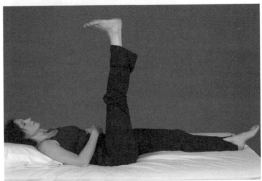

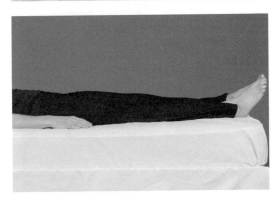

ROUNDHOUSE LEG KICK—LEFT LEG

- Lie with your arms at your sides and legs flat on the bed.

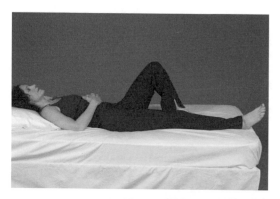

- Bend your left knee, keeping your foot flat on the bed, and then straighten your leg up toward the ceiling.

- Lower the leg across your body toward the right side of the bed, toes touching the bed if possible. (Let your hips and shoulders rotate to help your leg cross your body.)

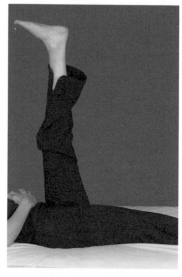

- Return your leg, hips, and shoulders to the starting position by bringing your leg back straight up toward the ceiling, then down on the bed.

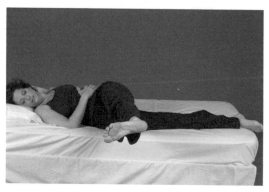

- Repeat three times.

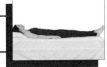

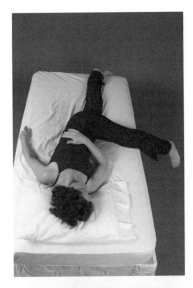

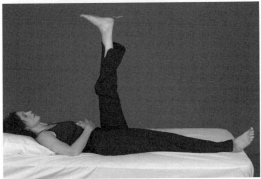

LEGS UPWARD STOMACH CRUNCH

- Start with your knees bent and feet flat on the bed.

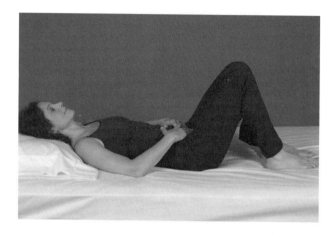

- Lift both legs toward the ceiling as much as you can (you may be more comfortable with your knees slightly bent).

- Using only your stomach muscles (not pulling with your neck or your arms), simultaneously raise your upper body and both hands toward your raised legs.

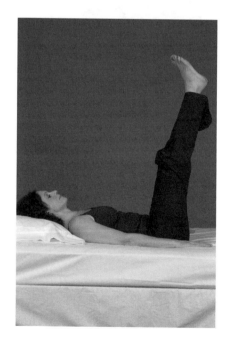

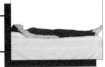

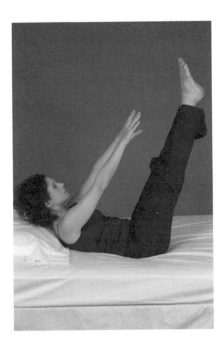

- Repeat crunch five times.

THE JAW DROP STRETCH

- Open and close your mouth widely, dropping your jaw for gentle stretching of your jaw muscles.

- Avoid overstretching your jaw.

- Repeat ten times.

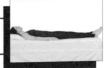

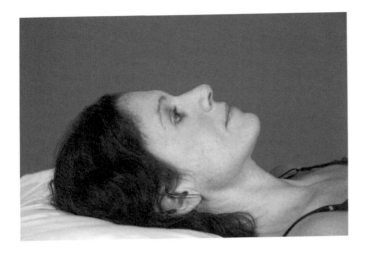

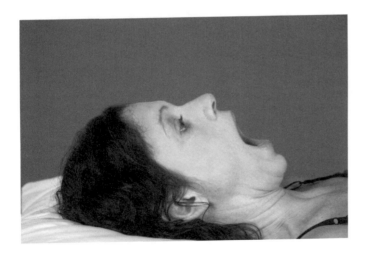

THE BICYCLE WITH PUNCHES

- Lie with your arms at your sides and legs flat on the bed.

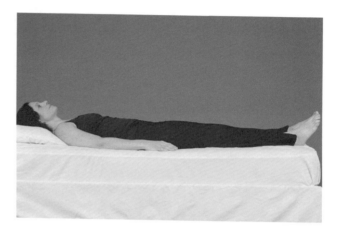

- Raise your legs and begin moving them as if you were pedaling a bicycle.

- Simultaneously, raise your upper body in a crunch-like position and begin throwing punches at your feet in sync with your leg movements.

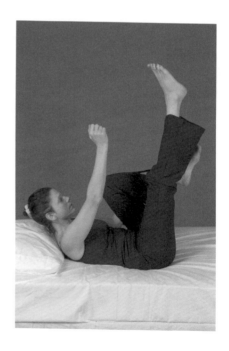

- Repeat ten times, hand punching and leg kicking five times each.

  TIP: *This exercise is terrific for self-defense.*

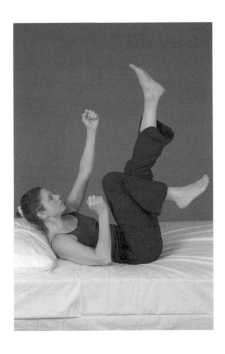

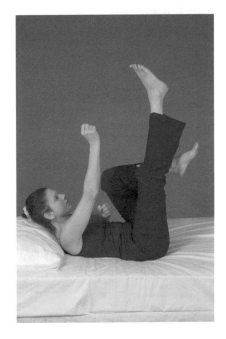

Dr. Genie's Modification:

With easy movements, alternate lifting to a comfortable height your left arm and left leg simultaneously, then your right arm and right leg simultaneously.

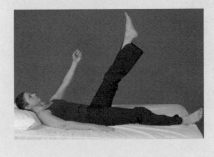

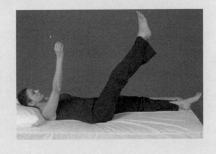

Summary of Photos for Exercises on Your Back

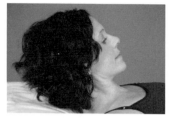

Raising Your Head
p. 18

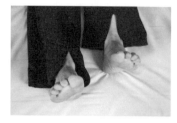

Alternate Leg Lengthener
p. 20

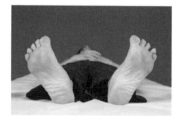

Ankle Circles
p. 22

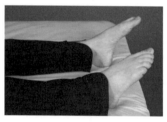

Pointing Feet and Toes
p. 24

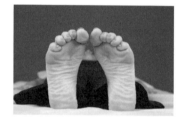

Toe Wiggling
p. 26

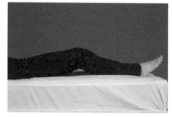

Knee Bounce, Thigh Flex
p. 28

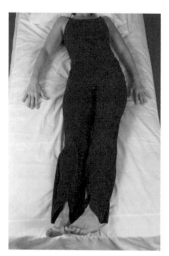

Hips Side to Side
p. 30

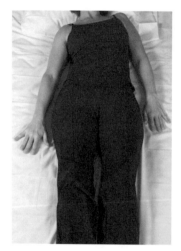

Arms-Shoulders Seesaw
p. 32

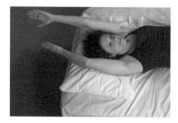

Arms Toward Headboard
p. 34

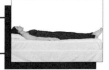

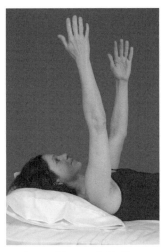

Arms Toward Ceiling
p. 36

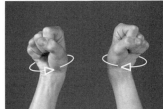
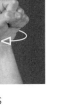

Wrist Circles
p. 38

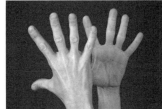

Finger Fling
p. 40

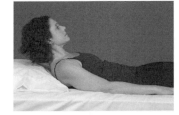

Minimal Crunch
p. 42

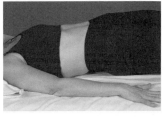

Modified Pelvic Tilt
p. 44

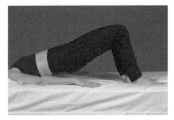

The Bridge
p. 46

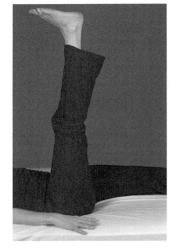

Karate Snap Kick—
Right Leg
p. 50

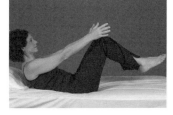

The Crunch
p. 52

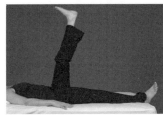

Karate Snap Kick—
Left Leg
p. 48

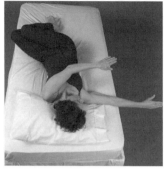
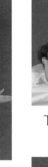

The Arm-Leg Switch
p. 54

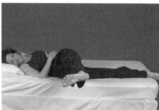

The Elbow-Knee Piston
p. 56

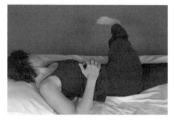

Roundhouse Leg
Kick—Right Leg
p. 58

Round House Leg Kick—
Left Leg
p. 60

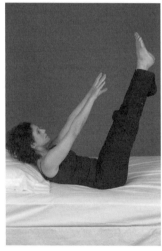

Legs Upward Stomach
Crunch
p. 62

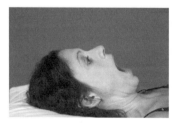

The Jaw Drop Stretch
p. 64

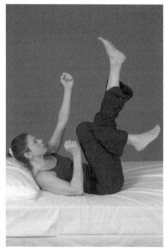

The Bicycle with Punches
p. 66

CHAPTER THREE

EXERCISES ON YOUR RIGHT SIDE

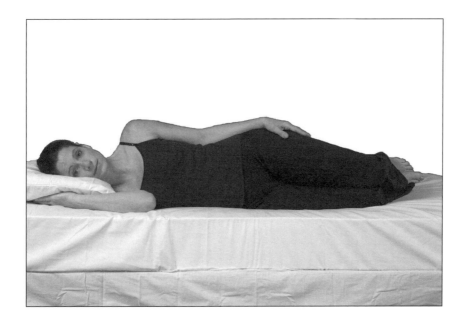

RAISING YOUR HEAD

- Lie on your side.

- Raise your head toward the ceiling (avoid straining your neck).

- Hold for two seconds.

- Lower your head back to the bed and hold for a count of two.

- Repeat ten times.

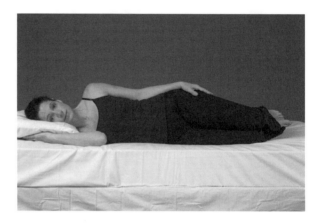

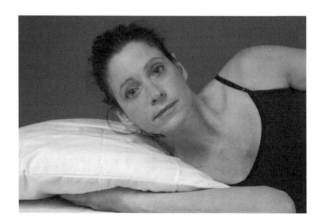

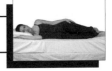

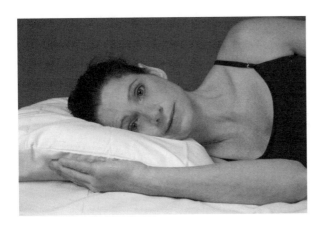

TIP: *For all exercises on your side, use of a thin pillow is optional. If you have neck problems, use a thin pillow to support your head and neck.*

SIDE LEG RAISES

- Start with your legs stacked, one leg on top of the other. (**Note:** The rest of the exercises on your right side start with the legs stacked.)

- Raise your left leg as high as you comfortably can toward the ceiling without rolling your hips.

- Hold for two seconds.

- Lower your left leg to the stacked position.

- Repeat five times.

Dr. Genie's Modification:

If you have lower back problems, bend your knees.

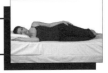

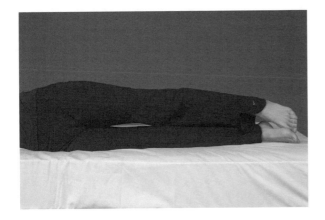

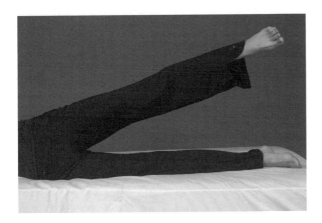

75

BOTTOM LEG, INNER THIGH TIGHTENER

- Raise your upper (left) leg from the stacked position and move it either forward or back, clearing your lower (right) leg for movement.

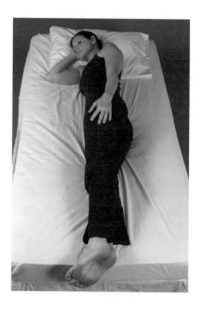

- Lift your lower (right) leg toward the ceiling.

- Repeat five times.

TIP: *The movement may be small, but raising the lower leg tightens and strengthens the inner thigh.*

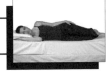

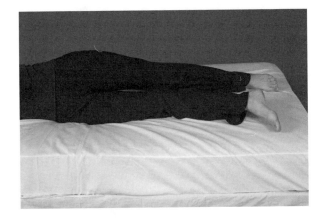

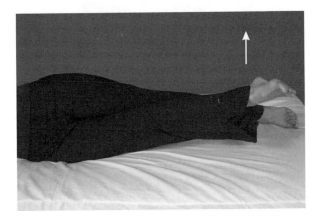

KNEE KICK

- Bring the knee of your left leg up toward your belly button.

- Return your leg back to the stacked position.

- Repeat five times.

  TIP: *Do this gently and slowly at first. As in all the exercises, increase speed and the number of repetitions as your muscles get conditioned.*

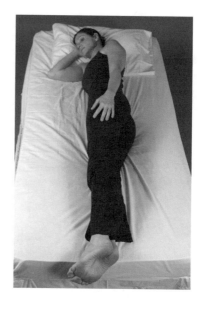

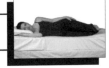

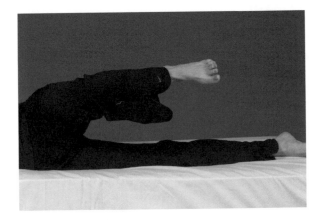

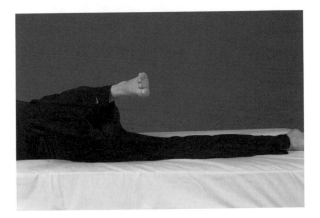

SIDE (OBLIQUES) STRENGTHENER

- Bend your left knee.

- Raise your upper body, exhaling while reaching your left arm toward your left leg.

- Lower your upper body back toward the bed (it need not go all the way down).

- Repeat three times.

  TIP: *Reach for your leg only as far as you can. Do not strain.*

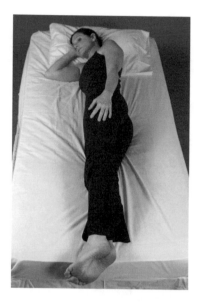

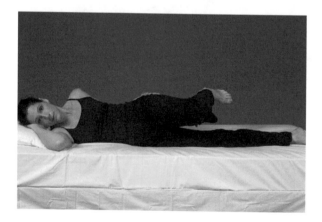

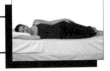

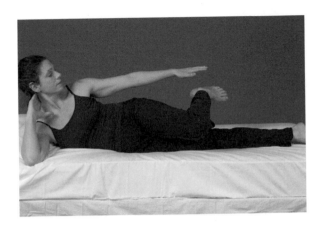

Dr. Genie's Modification:

Lift only the bent leg up and down. Omit the upper body movement.

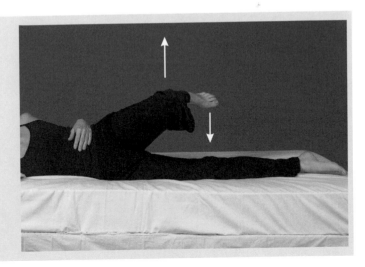

LEFT LEG REACHES BACK TOWARD LEFT HAND

- Bend your left leg backward, as if trying to touch your left foot to your buttocks.

- Reach your left hand back toward the foot of the bent leg.

- If you can, grasp your left ankle to help stretch the front leg muscle.

- Hold for three seconds.

- Repeat three times.

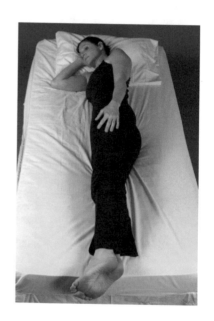

TIP: *Tighten your stomach muscles to protect your lower back. The left leg is doing most of the work here, giving a stretch to the front of your thigh. The amount of movement achieved depends upon your flexibility.*

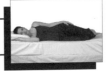

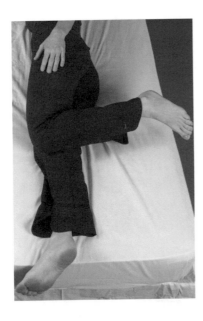

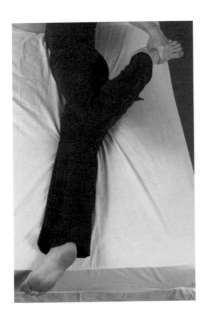

83

SIDE KICK

- Raise your left knee toward your belly button.

- Gently thrust your left leg toward the ceiling to a height you can manage.

- Bring your knee and leg back to the starting position.

- Repeat five times.

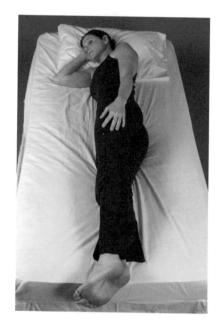

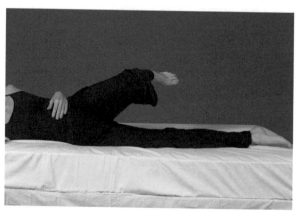

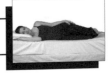

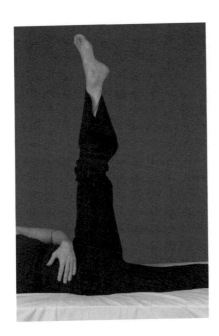

Summary of Photos for Exercises on Your Right Side

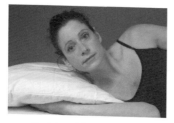

Raising Your Head
p. 72

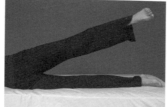

Side Leg Raises
p. 74

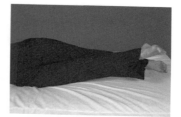

Bottom Leg, Inner Thigh
Tightener)
p. 76

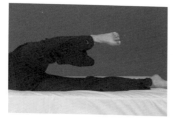

Knee Kick
p. 78

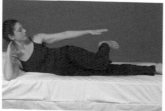

Side (Obliques)
Strengthener
p. 80

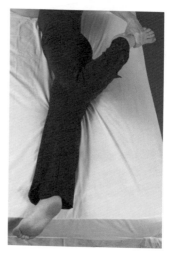

Left Leg Reaches Back
Toward Left Hand
p. 82

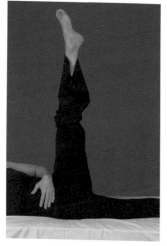

Side Kick
p. 84

CHAPTER FOUR

EXERCISES ON YOUR
LEFT SIDE

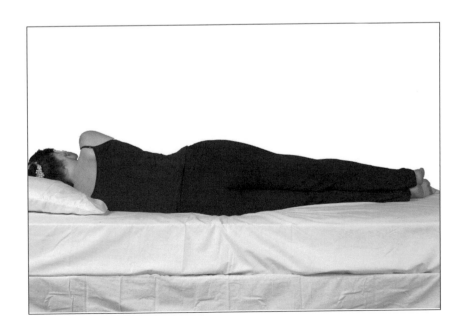

RAISING YOUR HEAD

- Lie on your side.

- Raise your head toward the ceiling (avoid straining your neck).

- Hold for two seconds.

- Lower your head back to the bed and hold for a count of two.

- Repeat ten times.

TIP: *For all exercises on your side, use of a thin pillow is optional. If you have neck problems, use a thin pillow to support your head and neck.*

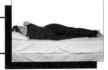

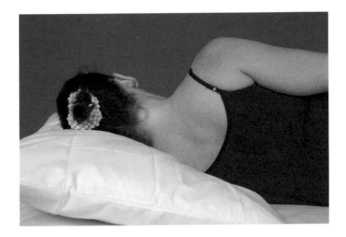

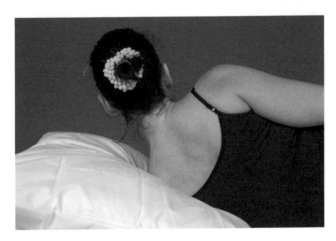

SIDE LEG RAISES

- Start with your legs stacked, one leg on top of the other. (**Note:** The rest of the exercises on your left side start with the legs stacked.)

- Raise your right leg as high as you comfortably can toward the ceiling without rolling your hips.

- Hold for two seconds.

- Lower your right leg to the stacked position.

- Repeat five times.

Dr. Genie's Modification:

If you have lower back problems, bend your knees.

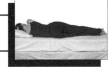

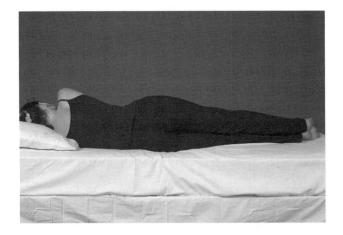

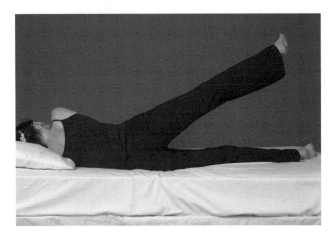

91

BOTTOM LEG, INNER THIGH TIGHTENER

- Raise your upper (right) leg from the stacked position and move it either forward or back, clearing your lower (left) leg for movement.

- Lift your lower (left) leg toward the ceiling.

- Repeat five times.

  TIP: *The movement may be small, but raising the lower leg tightens and strengthens the inner thigh.*

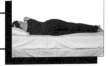

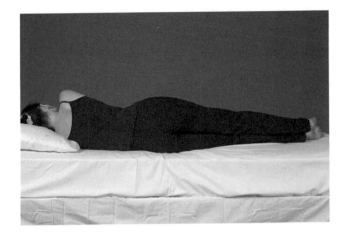

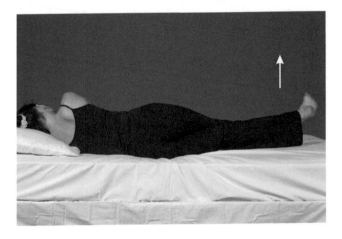

KNEE KICK

- Bring the knee of your right leg up toward your belly button.

- Return your leg back to the stacked position.

- Repeat five times.

    TIP: *Do this gently and slowly at first. As in all the exercises, increase speed and the number of repetitions as your muscles get conditioned.*

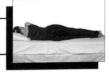

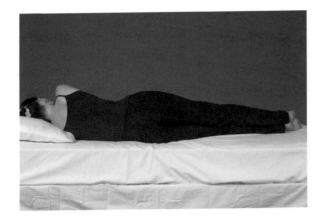

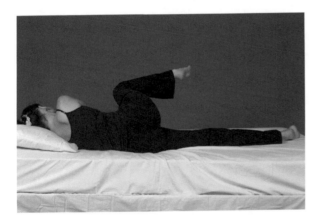

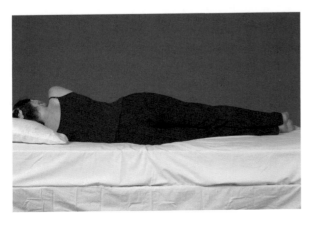

SIDE (OBLIQUES) STRENGTHENER

- Bend your right knee.

- Raise your upper body, exhaling while reaching your right arm toward your right leg.

- Lower your upper body back toward the bed (it need not go all the way down).

- Repeat three times.

  TIP: *Reach for your leg only as far as you can. Do not strain.*

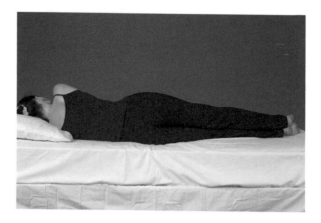

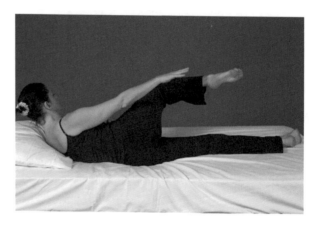

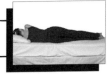

Dr. Genie's Modification:

Lift only the bent leg up and down. Omit the upper body movement.

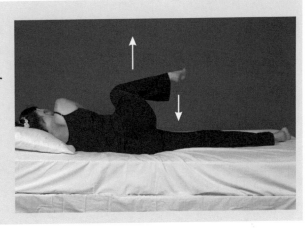

RIGHT LEG REACHES BACK TOWARD RIGHT HAND

- Bend your right leg backward, as if trying to touch your right foot to your buttocks.

- Reach your right hand back toward the foot of the bent leg.

- If you can, grasp your right ankle to help stretch the front leg muscle.

- Hold for three seconds.

- Repeat three times.

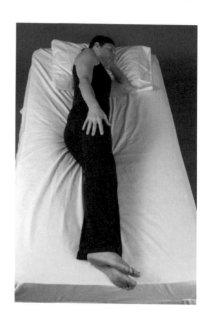

TIP: *Tighten your stomach muscles to protect your lower back. The right leg is doing most of the work here, giving a stretch to the front of your thigh. The amount of movement achieved depends upon your flexibility.*

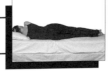

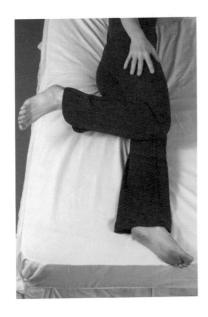

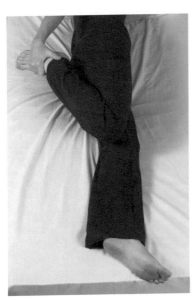

SIDE KICK

- Raise your right knee toward your belly button.

- Gently thrust your right leg toward the ceiling to a height you can manage.

- Bring your knee and leg back to the starting position.

- Repeat five times.

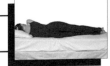

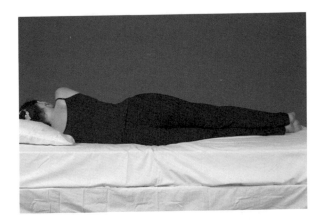

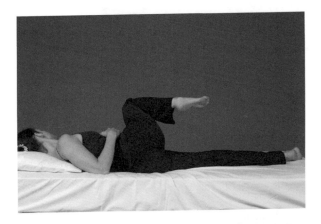

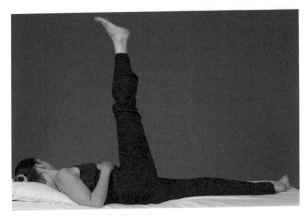

Summary of Photos for Exercises on Your Left Side

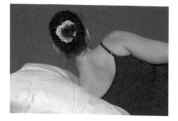

Raising Your Head
p. 88

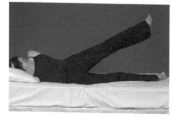

Side Leg Raises
p. 90

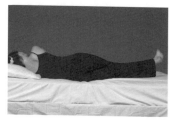

Bottom Leg, Inner Thigh
Tightener
p. 92

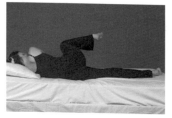

Knee Kick
p. 94

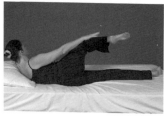

Side (Obliques)
Strengthener
p. 96

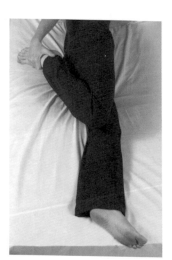

Right Leg Reaches Back
Toward Right Hand
p. 98

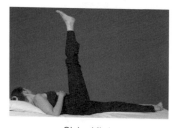

Side Kick
p. 100

CHAPTER FIVE

EXERCISES ON YOUR STOMACH

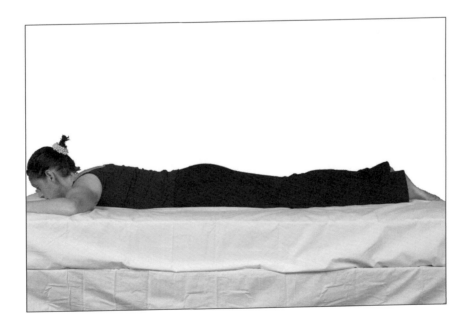

RAISING YOUR HEAD

- Lie on your stomach with your head facing downward on the bed.

- Gently lift your head and then place it back down.

- Repeat ten times.

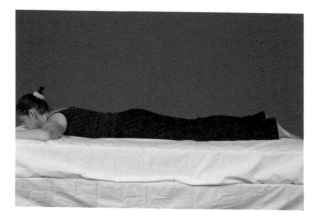

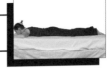

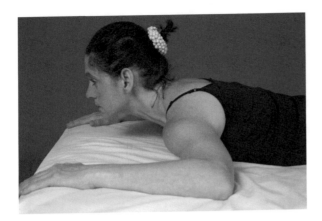

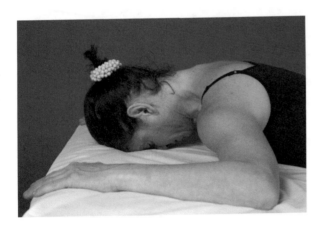

Dr. Genie's Modification:

If you are an older adult, or if you have a large stomach, you should place a pillow under your chest for comfort.

FLUTTER SWIM KICK

- With your chin and chest resting on the bed, alternately raise each leg off the bed in a swimmer's style flutter kick.

- Keep your legs straight and increase the height of your kicks for maximum glute tightening. Your pelvis should maintain contact with the bed.

- Kick fifteen times with each leg.

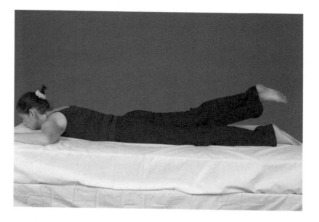

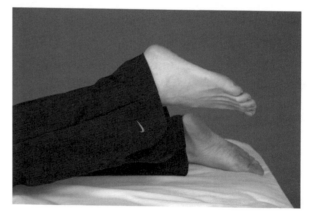

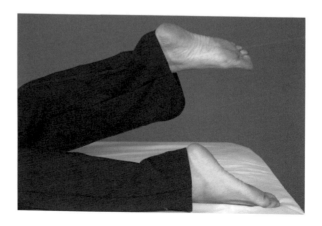

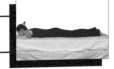

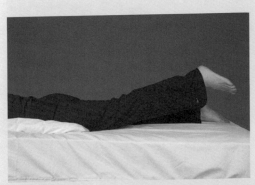

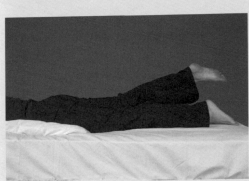

Dr. Genie's Modification:

If you have back pain, you should use a pillow under your hips. Stop this or any exercise if you experience shortness of breath.

FOREARM-SUPPORTED BODY LIFT

- Start with your fore-arms on the bed, hands near your shoulders.

- Using your chest and back muscles (and with forearms for support, like a tripod), lift your head and upper body simultaneously. Do not pull up with your neck.

- Hold for two seconds and return to the original position.

- Repeat five times.

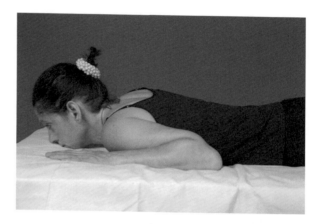

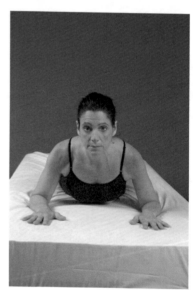

  TIP: *This is not a push-up, so your fore-arms are only for support as you lift your upper body.*

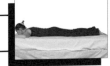

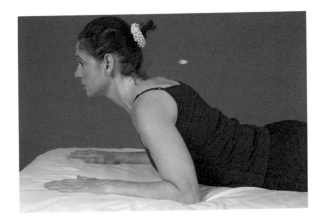

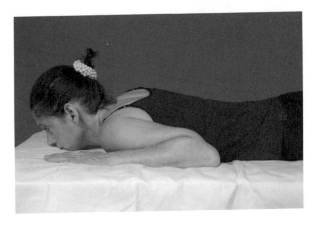

Dr. Genie's Modification:

Place a pillow under your hips.

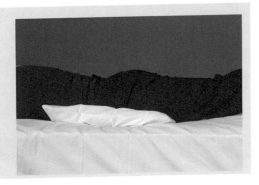

DOUBLE LEG DOLPHIN-STYLE KICK

- Start with your fore-
  arms on the bed,
  hands near your
  shoulders.

- Raise and then
  lower your legs
  together as if they
  were joined into
  one large swim fin.

- Repeat five times.

  TIP: *Keeping your legs
  straight is good for your
  glutes.*

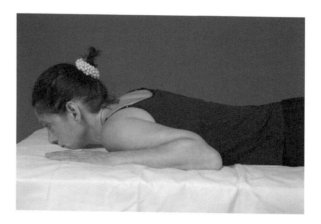

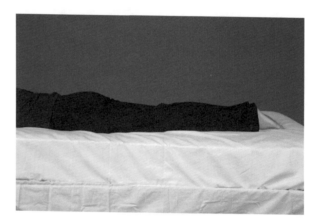

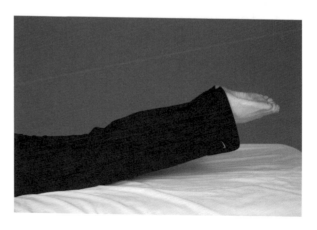

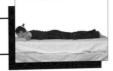

Dr. Genie's Modification:

Place a pillow under your hips. Remember to breathe evenly while performing this exercise.

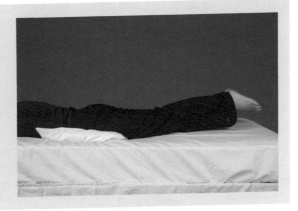

THE COBRA

- Start with your elbows bent and hands placed flat on the bed in line with your shoulders.

- Fully straighten your arms to lift your upper body while curving it back like a cobra.

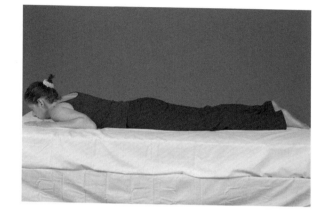

- If you cannot straighten your arms fully, go up as far as you can. (A soft mattress may affect your ability to get full extension.)

- Hold the up position for a few seconds and then return to the starting position.

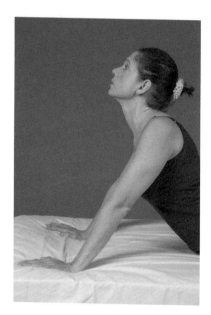

- Repeat two times.

TIP: *Try this exercise using deeper breathing.*

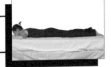

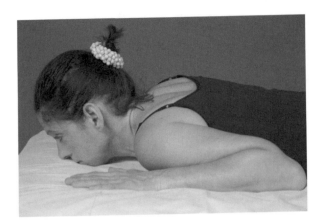

Dr. Genie's Modification:

If you have shoulder or lower back problems, do the cobra using your forearms to lift your upper body.

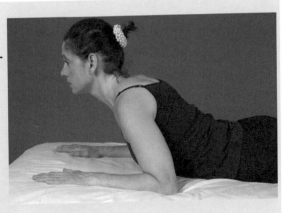

113

THE LOCUST

- Start with your arms at your sides and your hands slightly under your thighs.

- Slowly lift both legs simultaneously as you tighten your buttocks for support.

- Hold the up position for a few seconds and then bring your legs back down.

- Repeat two times.

TIP: *Try this exercise using deeper breathing.*

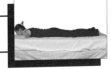

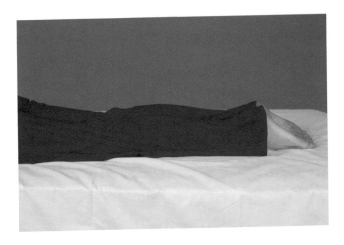

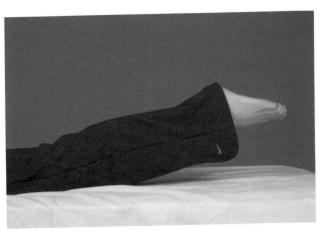

Dr. Genie's Modification:

Don't raise the legs. Just tighten your buttocks.

THE MODIFIED BOW

- While on your stomach, raise your legs and upper body simultaneously.

- Reach back with your arms as if trying to touch your raised feet.

- Hold the up position for a few seconds and then return to the starting position.

- Repeat two times.

TIP: *Try this exercise using deeper breathing.*

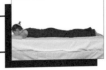

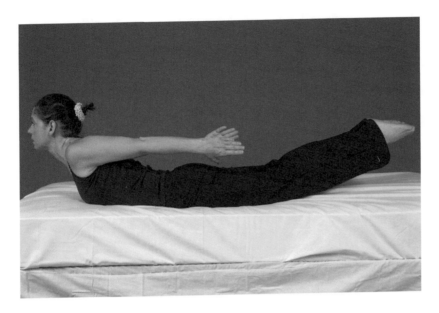

SWIMMING IN BED

- Just as if you are in a pool or the ocean, do a swim stroke in bed known as the Australian crawl (for many of us, what we do may more closely resemble the dog paddle).

- For nonswimmers, that means reaching forward alternately with each arm while doing flutter kicks.

- Repeat twenty times, counting each arm movement as one.

TIP: *You don't need to raise your arms off the bed. You can just slide them forward as you reach out with the alternating arm movements.*

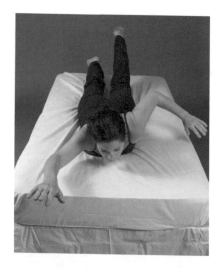

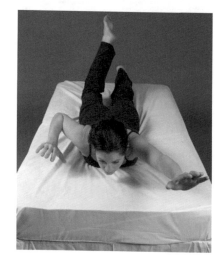

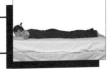

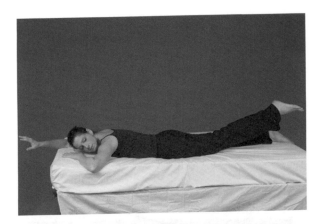

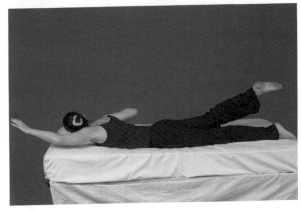

Dr. Genie's Modification:

Use a pillow under your hips. Remember to breathe evenly.

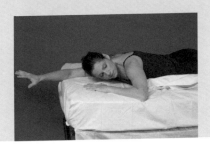

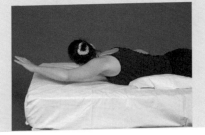

OPTIONAL REPEAT: THE BRIDGE

TIP: *Exercises on your stomach can place some stress on the lower back. The bridge helps to relax the lower back. For that, we suggest doing a few additional bridges.*

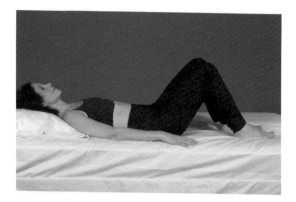

- Start on your back with your knees bent and feet flat on the bed. Place your arms at your sides.

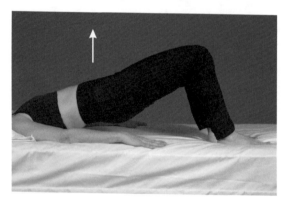

- Tighten the buttock muscles as you lift your pelvis toward the ceiling until pelvis is in line with your thighs.

- Come back down to the bed gently.

- Repeat five times.

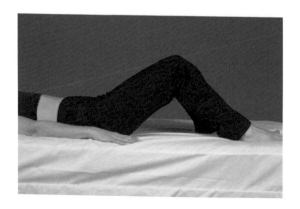

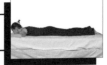

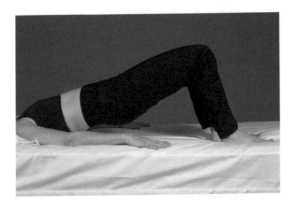

Dr. Genie's Modification

If you have back or knee problems, place your feet further from your buttocks and raise your pelvis only to a comfortable level.

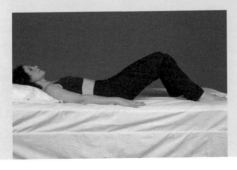 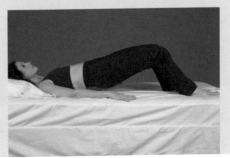

Summary of Exercises on Your Stomach

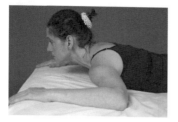

Raising Your Head
p. 104

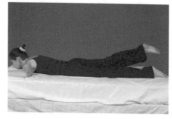

Flutter Swim Kick
p. 106

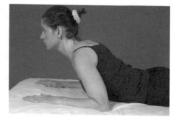

Forearm-Supported
Body Lift
p. 108

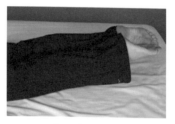

Double Leg
Dolphin-Style Kick
p. 110

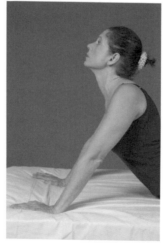

The Cobra
p. 112

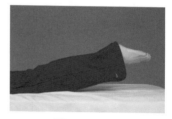

The Locust
p. 114

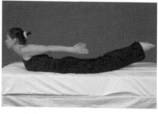

The Modified Bow
p. 116

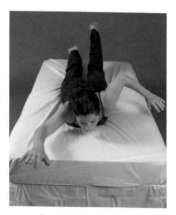

Swimming in Bed
p. 118

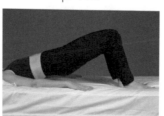

OPTIONAL REPEAT:
The Bridge
p. 120

CHAPTER SIX

SUMMARY OF ALL THE EXERCISES

After you have practiced the exercises for a while, you may remember them well enough to start doing them without always referring to the book. If you are like the two of us, you will probably get some of them out of order. Ted says it happens to him often, even after all the years he has been doing them. Remember that you should always make exercising in bed a stress-free experience. Don't let yourself worry if your body is not exactly in the position that you see in the photos. Don't be overly concerned about the number of repetitions you choose to do or the speed at which you do them. This is your bed, your special place of rest and recuperation, and you should feel in control of your decision-making while there. Create an exercise level that is comfortable for you. Vary your practice as you like, sometimes doing one segment of the exercises, sometimes another, and sometimes all of them in sequence.

We have found increased body strength, flexibility, calmness, and ease of sleep to be the benefits of these routines. If you do these exercises regularly, we believe you will find that to be true for you, too. You will be more likely to achieve these results if you stay relaxed while doing the exercises. Our best wishes for your good health and added fitness.

Here's a quick summary of all the exercise for easy reference:

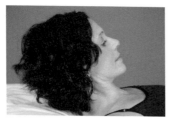

Raising Your Head
p. 18

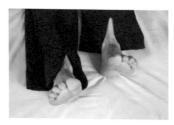

Alternate Leg Lengthener
p. 20

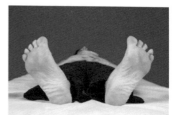

Ankle Circles
p. 22

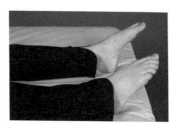

Pointing Feet and Toes
p. 24

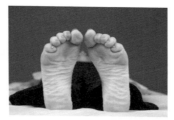

Toe Wiggling
p. 26

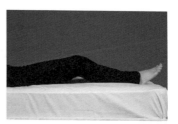

Knee Bounce, Thigh Flex
p. 28

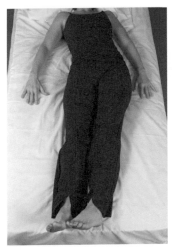

Hips Side to Side
p. 30

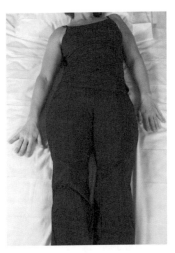

Arms-Shoulders Seesaw
p. 32

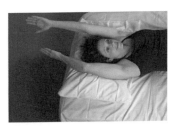

Arms Toward Headboard
p. 34

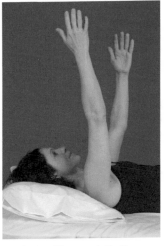

Arms Toward Ceiling
p. 36

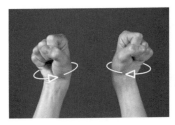

Wrist Circles
p. 38

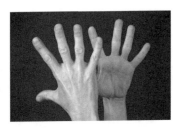

Finger Fling
p. 40

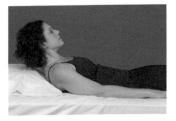

Minimal Crunch
p. 42

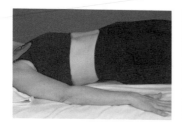

Modified Pelvic Tilt
p. 44

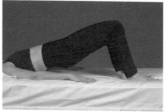

The Bridge
p. 46

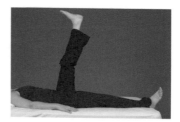

Karate Snap Kick—
Left Leg
p. 48

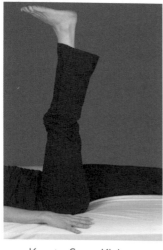

Karate Snap Kick—
Right Leg
p. 50

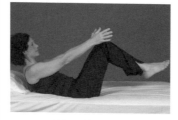

The Crunch
p. 52

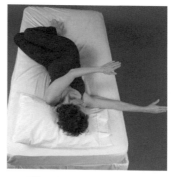

The Arm-Leg Switch
p. 54

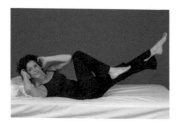

The Elbow-Knee Piston
p. 56

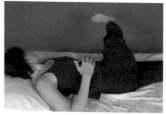

Roundhouse Leg
Kick—Right Leg
p. 58

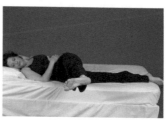

Roundhouse Leg
Kick—Left Leg
p. 60

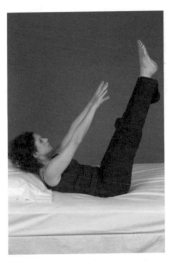

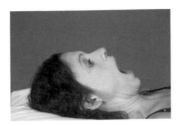

The Jaw Drop Stretch
p. 64

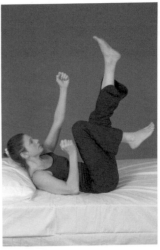

Legs Upward Stomach
Crunch
p. 62

The Bicycle with Punches
p. 66

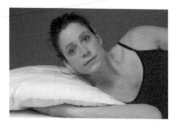

Raising Your Head
p. 72

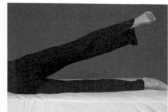

Side Leg Raises
p. 74

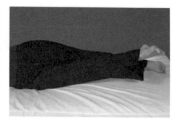

Bottom Leg, Inner Thigh
Tightener
p. 76

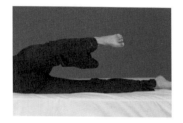

Knee Kick
p. 78

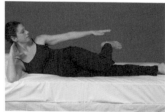

Side (Obliques)
Strengthener
p. 80

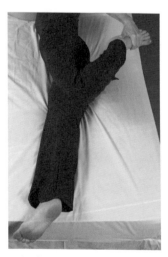

Left Leg Reaches Back
Toward Left Hand
p. 82

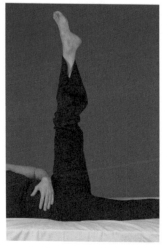

Side Kick
p. 84

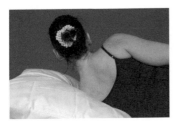

Raising Your Head
p. 88

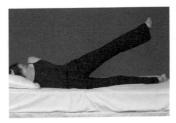

Side Leg Raises
p. 90

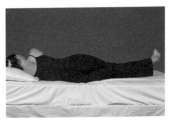

Bottom Leg, Inner Thigh
Tightener
p. 92

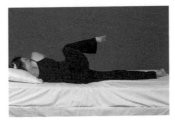

Knee Kick
p. 94

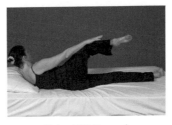

Side (Obliques)
Strengthener
p. 96

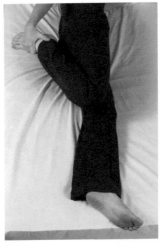

Right Leg Reaches Back
Toward Right Hand
p. 98

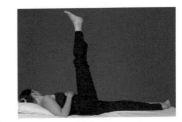

Side Kick
p. 100

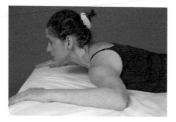
Raising Your Head
p. 104

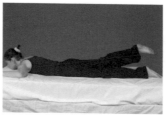
Flutter Swim Kick
p. 106

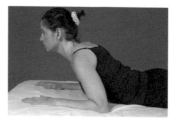
Forearm Supported
Body Lift
p. 108

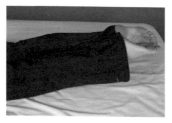
Double Leg Dolphin-Style
Kick
p. 110

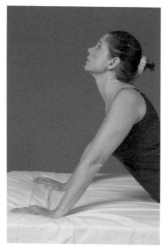
The Cobra
p. 112

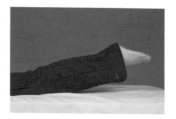
The Locust
p. 114

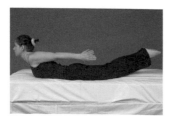
The Modified Bow
p. 116

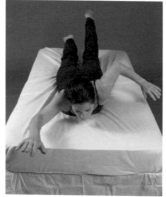
Swimming in Bed
p. 118

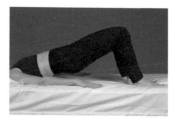
OPTIONAL REPEAT:
The Bridge
p. 120

Other New Harbinger Titles

Eating Mindfully, Item 3503, $13.95

TriEngergetics, Item 4453, $15.95

Eating Wisely for Hormonal Balance, Item 3732, $16.95

Living Beyond Your Pain, Item 4097, $19.95

The Trigger Point Therapy Workbook, 2nd ed, Item 3759, $19.95

The Frozen Shoulder Workbook, Item 447X, $18.95

Pilates for Fragile Backs, Item 4666, $18.95

Solid to the Core, Item 4305, $14.95

Move Your Body, Tone Your Mood, Item 2752, $17.95

The Ten Hidden Barriers to Weight Loss, Item 3244, $11.95

The MS Workbook, Item 3902, $19.95

Fibromyalgia and Chronic Myofascial Pain Syndrome, 2nd ed,
Item 2388 $19.95

available at bookstores nationwide

To order, call toll free, **1-800-748-6273,** or visit our online bookstore at **www.newharbinger.com**. Have your Visa or Mastercard number ready.

Prices subject to change without notice.